...ING FOR ...QUET SPORTS

Christopher M. Norris

A&C BLACK, LONDON

First published in 2008 by
A & C Black Publishers Ltd
38 Soho Square
London W1D 3HB
www.acblack.com

ISBN 978 1 408106 95 2

A CIP catalogue record for this book is available from the British Library.

This book is produced using paper from wood grown in managed, sustainable forests. It is natural, renewable and recyclable. The logging and manufacturing processes conform to the environmental regulations of the country of origin.

Typeset in Din Light by Palimpsest Book Production Limited, Grangemouth, Stirlingshire

Cover image © Corbis
Inside photography © Grant Pritchard, except pages 2, 6, 60, 80, 90 © Shutterstock
Illustrations © Jeff Edwards

Printed and bound in China by South China Printing Co.

CONTENTS

Acknowledgements

My thanks go to Susie Gale, Victoria Jones, Jean Nadin, Madge Slater and Suzanne Hattersley, who modelled for the exercises.

1

Introduction

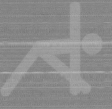

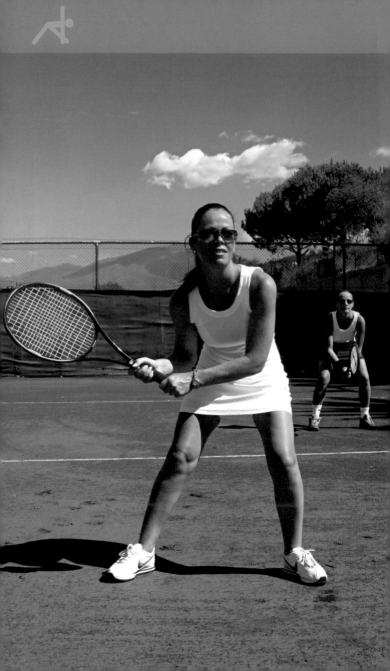

1. Introduction

Why stretch?

Stretching is an important part of any training programme. It has two principal effects: it can help to reduce the likelihood of injury, and it also works to improve your performance. Injury prevention and performance enhancement are features close to the hearts of many racquet sportsmen and women, and for this reason stretching should become part of your exercise programme.

As with any sport, racquet sports place stress on particular areas of the body. The hips, upper body and back come under considerable strain – the hips are turned for every movement on court, so they should be as flexible as possible. The back also takes a great deal of strain, for example bending to reach shots and reaching to serve or take an overhead volley. Your shoulders also need to be well prepared for the demands of your service action. As well as these core parts of the body, wrists, elbows, calves and ankles are placed under particular strain on court.

Most racquet sports players feel that time away from their sport is time wasted, but the reverse is actually true. Maintaining a regular stretching programme is a wise investment for your sporting future.

How to use this book

You can use this book in a number of ways. If you wish, you can use the exercises in Chapter 3 as a three-phase programme, over nine or ten weeks. If you follow this programme, with each phase building on the previous one, you should find that you gain in flexibility over that period, and so improve your performance and help reduce your risk of injury.

If you prefer, however, you can use the exercises to design a programme specifically to meet your needs – whether you know you have a weak point, or are trying to get back to fitness from an injury, or want to build particular stretching exercises into your overall fitness programme.

In Chapter 2, we look first at the importance of warming up – whether before stretching or before playing – and the best ways of going about this. Second, we aim to help you work out how flexible you are at the outset – this may help you to decide whether you want to improve your flexibility overall, or whether to focus particularly on certain areas. The chart on pages 13–17 will help you measure this. We then discuss briefly the different types of stretches and how and when to use them, and finally what to expect in terms of improvement if you follow the stretching programme.

Chapter 3 contains the exercises themselves, divided into three sections – beginner, intermediate and advanced. Each section begins with a note on how to use the exercises. As we are all different, many of the exercises include variations and important points to note, which often relate to your safety. You can use the training log (Chapter 5) if you wish to keep a record of your progress.

Chapter 4 looks at the injuries most common among racquet players, how to deal with them, and particularly at how to get back to fitness using stretching exercises. Useful terms are explained in Chapter 6.

All the exercises suggested in this book can be performed either at home or in the gym. Some can be used before you go on court as part of your warm-up, but remember stretching as part of a warm-up must be gentle – suitable stretches are listed on page 11. The majority, however, should be used in a separate session.

Several of the advanced exercises are designed to be used with a partner, as there are specific benefits to be gained from stretching with the aid of someone else. If you don't have a training partner, you will still be able to do the exercises, but with a partner you are able to relax much more into the stretch.

The three-phase programme is designed to improve your flexibility and target muscles appropriate to your individual needs. During the programme you will come to identify certain exercises which feel particularly useful, and these can become part of your general training programme in the long-term.

2

Before you start

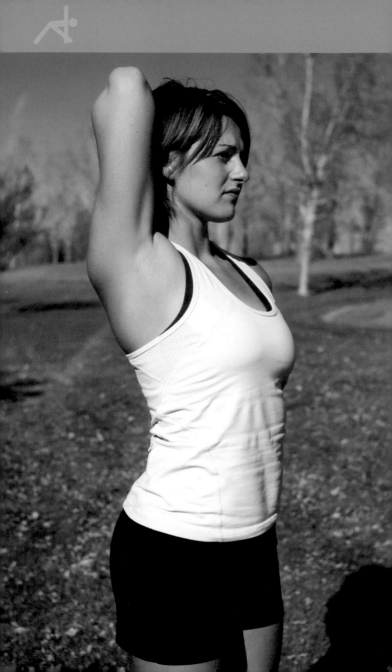

Equipment

Before you begin stretching, make sure you have the following:
- Sufficient space to perform the exercises – if you are practising at home you may need to move furniture
- A non-slip mat such as a yoga mat which is springy
- Loose clothing which will not restrict your movements or ride up
- A towel to dry down so you don't get cold.

Warming up

Before we start stretching (or playing), we need to warm up. Stretching on cold and unprepared muscle is not very effective, and in some cases can be quite dangerous. Make sure you wear layered clothing: for example, shorts and T-shirt underneath and fleecy bottoms and top to cover up. Begin covered and as you feel warm, you can peel layers off. When you stretch your legs, put your top back on, and when you stretch your arms take the top off and put your bottoms on.

Any warm-up has effects in three areas: the circulation, the body tissues and the mind.

The good . . .

Circulatory effects
These are especially important for the heart. If you progress quickly from rest, when your heart rate is quite low, to strenuous exercise, when your heart is pumping rapidly, your heart is put under too much stress. In fact, scientists in the early 1970s showed that such rapid changes in the heart rate could actually cause it to miss beats (the medical term for this is an ectopic beat). This can be very serious in an older person or someone with a history of heart or circulation problems.

Any intense exercise done from a cold start can be potentially harmful, and this was the case with squash when it first became popular. Because it was seen as a 'social' sport by many, people often started the game in poor physical condition, having done little exercise since leaving school many years before. The combination of poor fitness and lack of knowledge about exercise had serious consequences for some – a point grasped by the media at the time, to the detriment of the game.

Body tissue effects

These effects occur when the tissues you are going to stretch heat up. At any one time, your body actually has more blood vessels than it needs for the amount of blood they carry. This means that should all the blood vessels open at once, the blood will drop down towards your feet – exactly what happens when you faint! To prevent this, the body only opens up the blood vessels that it needs. After a heavy meal, the blood vessels to your stomach and intestines are opened; but during exercise these are closed, and those to the working muscles are opened instead. You need to make sure, then, that the right blood vessels are opened, and that is the function of a warm-up – to shunt fresh blood into the tissue you are about to stretch. Blood is warm, and as it warms the tissues they become more pliable, just like putty.

Mental effects

Mental effects relate to two things – arousal level and mental rehearsal. We all have times when we feel drowsy, with heavy eyelids. Everything feels like hard work, and this is because our arousal level is low. But if someone creeps up behind you and suddenly claps their hands, you jump and your heart rate soars. Now, with arousal level increased, you are ready for anything. This is what a warm-up can do – it focuses your attention on exercise and increases your arousal level.

Another effect of warming up, and one which is probably more important within the field of stretching, is mental rehearsal. This becomes vital where complex skilled actions are needed, such as coordination and stretch combined. This is seen in complex shots such as twisting to take a backhand off one foot.

At the end of any period of exercise you will have practised a number of movements which are very familiar to you – you know which parts of the body to move and how far to move them. However, in the days between workouts you may forget the skills involved in the exercise. If you go straight into a skilled exercise, expecting to perform it as well as you did during your last workout, you will find that you are not able to do so. You may wobble dangerously, and will increase the chances of pulling a muscle.

In this case, you can use a warm-up to remind yourself of the movement. You can do this with a couple of simple actions and then build up the complexity. In tennis, for example, you might perform a series of forehand and backhand actions without hitting the ball and then progress to striking the ball at low intensity before building up.

. . . and the bad

The idea of a warm-up is to prepare you for exercise. It should help you to perform the exercises better, and reduce the chances of getting injured. Normally this is the case, but in some instances a warm-up can be detrimental.

Damage often occurs when extreme stretching is used as part of a warm-up. This is because, after extreme stretching, your muscles are tired and aching, and so you are more likely to be injured if, for example, you make a sudden and powerful movement. If your muscles are fatigued, you will also not be able to perform as well in a sport which involves heavy muscle work – if you were to do a high jump, for example. Stretching your leg muscles until they really ache will mean that you can't jump as high.

This is really common sense, but it is important to differentiate between the two types of stretching – maintenance and developmental – which we will cover below.

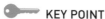

> ⌐○━ **KEY POINT**
> A warm-up should make you sweat lightly, and rehearse
> the actions you are about to use in the sport.

Practical warm-up

So, how do we warm up? Well, a good warm-up should:
- take your joints and muscles through their normal degree of movement (range of motion);
- increase your pulse enough to make you sweat very lightly.

If you miss out some joints, or don't sweat at all, your warm-up is not intense enough (too easy), but if you sweat profusely or end up with aching muscles your warm-up is too intense (too hard).

Let's take a brief look at a typical warm-up before a game and also before a stretching routine.

Before a game
- Begin with a slow walk, building up the speed to a power walk forwards, backwards and sideways to mimic the changing directions of racquet sports.
- Slowly circle your arms, taking two or three movements before you reach right overhead.
- Once you have done this for two to three minutes, build to a slow jog, using small, light steps, again in multiple directions.
- Continue this until you feel yourself sweating lightly.

This 5–10 minute warm-up takes care of the circulatory and body tissue elements. To warm up psychologically you will need to use movement rehearsal, and this is best done by performing an exercise at a lower intensity. Before a game, use your racquet to perform free actions (ie. not hitting a ball) for 5–10 repetitions. Use forehand, backhand, volley and serving actions, but at a much slower pace.

Before a stretching routine

Once you have performed your jogging action described opposite, you are then ready to move onto your stretching programme. Build up gradually, making sure you don't stretch too far, too fast. Try this progression, performing two repetitions of each movement:

- Move at 50–60 per cent of your motion range to begin with (see box).
- Rest and increase this range to 80–90 per cent for the second set.
- Only stretch fully (100–110 per cent) when sure that you are fully warm.

Remember that you don't need to stretch to extreme levels with every session.

Stretching to warm up

When you are warming up using stretching, you should take your joint through its near maximum comfortable range, but no further (don't push it!). This is still stretching, of course, because if you have been sitting at your office desk all day, your muscles are stiff. You then need to stretch to your full range to get rid of the stiffness and lengthen your body tissues to their full, comfortable level. When you were sitting at work, you may have used only 20 per cent of your potential stretch.

Intensive (also known as developmental) stretching takes this range further: you move to 100 per cent of your range and then try to increase from this (100–110 per cent). Now you are actually trying to make your tissues more flexible that they have been before. *The golden rule is not to use intensive stretching before sport or as part of a warm-up.* Instead, you should warm up in order to stretch.

Putting stretches in a warm-up is fine providing you are using lower levels of stretching – perhaps 50–60 per cent of your movement range. Any more is counterproductive, as it will leave you sore and so affect your performance.

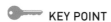

Checking your flexibility

Before you stretch it is helpful to record your current level of flexibility – how far you can actually stretch now. Why? Because this will be your baseline, the starting point against which you can measure your progress. If you don't know how flexible you were to begin with, you will often fail to see any progress in your stretching, because that progress will actually be quite slow. If you have nothing to measure progress against, it is easy to lose heart and become demotivated.

The other important reason to measure your flexibility is to find out whether your physique is balanced. Muscle imbalance is common, and occurs when some of your muscles are tight and when others are quite flexible. This is often brought about either by your job or by sport. In your job, if you sit hunched over a desk, you can easily become round-shouldered. This is a good example of muscle imbalance – your chest muscles are often tight, but your upper back muscles in contrast may be lax and too flexible. If you simply stretch all your muscles, you will certainly become more flexible, but your physique will still be imbalanced.

The chart on pages 13–17 shows some simple tests, which you can use to measure and record your current flexibility. Following a warm-up, you should perform each of these tests, holding the fully stretched position for 10 seconds. Pull into the position slowly, with no bouncing movements. Measure your scores, and record them on the chart (make a photocopy if you do not want to mark your book). Your measurement will give you a score of same as, less than or more than the average, and you may find that this varies between exercises. Some may be poor, some good, and this shows that muscle imbalance is present.

The score is for your guidance only – your individual measurement is actually more important as it represents your baseline measure, the one which you will be comparing against. You can retest your flexibility using this chart every week throughout the stretching programme to monitor your progress.

Testing your flexibility

Tick the box that corresponds to your movement range, following the guidelines given for each test. Recheck each week.

- Remember to warm up first.
- Hold each stretch for three seconds before measuring.
- Do not bounce into the movement.
- Average values vary with body size and type.

Test	Less	Average	More
Keep your straight leg on the floor and pull your bent knee towards your chest	knee more than 15 cm from ribcage	knee 10–15 cm from ribcage	knee to ribcage
Place the soles of your feet together and press your knees downwards towards the floor	more than 15 cm from floor	15 cm from floor	less than 15 cm from floor

Test	Less	Average	More
Keep your knees locked and reach forwards towards your toes	more than 15 cm from toes	10–15 cm from toes	touching toes
Bend your lower leg up to your chest and hold still; lower your top leg towards the ground	above horizontal	horizontal	below horizontal
Stand 0.5 m from a wall. Lean forwards, keeping your feet flat on the floor and knees locked	more than 60 degrees	60 degrees	less than 60 degrees
Keep your forehead and chest on the ground and lift your arms upwards	less than 15 cm	15–20 cm	more than 20 cm

Test	Less	Average	More
Reach behind your back and try to grip the fingers of the opposite hand	fingers more than 15 cm apart	fingers 10–15 cm apart	fingers touching
Keep your arms straight and try to cross them over as far as possible	cross at wrist	cross at elbow	cross at upper arm
Keep your foot flat on a stool and press your knee towards the wall	more than 50 degrees	40–50 degrees	less than 40 degrees
Keep your knees together and bent to 90 degrees. Allow your heels to drop downwards	less than 70 degrees	70–90 degrees	more than 90 degrees

Test	Less	Average	More
Lock your arms flat out and measure the distance between the top of your pelvis and the floor	more than 15 cm	15–10 cm	less than 10 cm
Keeping your arms flat on the floor, twist your trunk to allow your knees to lower towards the floor	more than 10 cm from floor	up to 10 cm	0 cm
Keep the small of your back against the chair back and flex your spine (not your hips) as much as possible	fingers to mid-shin	fingers to floor	hand flat to floor
Keeping your feet flat and knees locked, reach down the side of your leg without leaning forwards or backwards	fingers above knee	fingers to knee	fingers below knee

Test	Less	Average	More
Keep both legs straight and flex one hip as far as possible	less than 90 degrees	90 degrees	more than 90 degrees
Push your legs apart while keeping the small of the back flat and your legs straight	less than 90 degrees between legs	90 degrees	more than 90 degrees
Keep your knees together and flex one knee as far as possible	heel more than 10 cm from buttock	heel 5–10 cm from buttock	heel to buttock
Keeping your knees and ankles together throughout, slowly sit back on your heels. Measure the distance between the top of the foot and the ground	more than 5 cm	up to 5 cm	flat

Types of stretching and how to use them

There are many different stretching methods available, but we will use the three most common types – static, dynamic, and tensing and releasing the muscle before stretching, known as contract–relax (CR). All are useful in helping to improve flexibility. The chart on page 26 shows which types of stretching can be used with the exercises in this programme. Further details are shown in the exercise section.

Static stretching

With static stretching you take your limb to the point where you begin to feel tight, and hold this position. This is the sort of flexibility used in yoga. As the position is held, your tissues are allowed to lengthen gradually, and naturally occurring muscle reflexes help the muscle to relax. This is the most common stretch we will use. All the exercises in phase I and most of those in phases II and III are static stretches.

Static stretching is a particularly safe method. However, because the position may be held for some time, the exercise position must be comfortable and well supported. If you wobble, the stretch may be jerked further, and this is quite dangerous. Lying or sitting on a mat are good positions for static stretches, but kneeling or standing on one leg are not.

Once you have achieved the right position, you need to concentrate on breathing out and 'sighing', because this will allow your muscles to relax further. Hold the stretched position initially for five seconds. Release the stretch and rest for 10–20 seconds to allow blood to flow back into the muscle, and then repeat the stretch. After three sessions of this stretching pattern, increase the holding time to 20–30 seconds, but still perform three repetitions.

After you have been using this stretching pattern for 10–14 days you can extend it to perform five repetitions, holding each for 30 seconds. When the stretch is released after each rep, release the muscle tension slowly, without allowing the tissues to 'spring' back. Recoil of this type can be painful.

The timing stated is for general guidance only. When you stretch, if you feel that holding for 30 seconds is too much, then just release the stretch. We all have off days. One day you might want to stretch more intensely and hold the stretch for longer, while on another day you might want to take it easy. It is more important to listen to your body and respond to its needs than to adhere rigorously to a set time frame.

 KEY POINT
With static stretching make sure you choose a stable body position and try to relax into the movement.

Dynamic stretching

Dynamic stretching simply means stretching while moving. For this type of stretching you end up in more or less the same position as with static stretching, but the idea is to move into this position in a controlled fashion. With dynamic stretching, you are using coordination and what is known as 'muscle sequencing' that is, one muscle working after another in a specific order. This can be very helpful in sport, where a dynamic stretch can begin to rehearse a sports action.

To illustrate the difference between static and dynamic stretching, let's take as an example an overhead shot. As you reach up and back with your racquet, your shoulder and arm muscles are stretched. When you take the shot, you throw your arm forward through a combination of recoil of the stretched muscles and contraction – the two forces combined give what's technically called a 'ballistic action'.

You can perform a static stretch for the front of the shoulder by standing side on to a wall and reaching your arm horizontally to touch the wall. To perform a dynamic stretch, simply use the same action, but grip a gym band or pulley fastened behind you at shoulder level. Pull forwards against the band, and then allow it to pull your arm backwards in a slow and controlled manner.

The key point with dynamic stretching is to maintain control throughout, and to never allow the action to become so rapid that you risk injury. Normally, a total movement in dynamic stretching should take about 10–15 seconds. If the action speeds up so that it only takes two–three seconds, the chances are that it is too fast – you should stop, rest, and begin again at a slower pace.

 KEY POINT
Dynamic stretching is stretching with movement.
It works several muscle groups in sequence.

Contract–relax

Contract–relax (CR) is a form of intense stretching designed to get the maximum stretch by using muscle reflexes. After you tense a muscle – a so-called *isometric* contraction – the muscle relaxes slightly so that its firmness (tone) is less tense than before. We use this fact in CR stretching. First we contract (tense) the muscle, then hold it for two to five seconds, and then relax. During the relaxation period, we stretch.

Nearly all the static stretches that we use in this programme can be converted to CR stretches if you want to take the stretch slightly further. This would be appropriate only after you have practised a stretch for several training sessions, or if you are used to stretching in general and would classify yourself as stretching at an advanced level.

Let's use a common hamstring stretch as an example. Lie on your back on the floor and lift your right leg, keeping it straight. Grasp your leg around your thigh and gently pull your straight leg towards you. Hold this position, breathing normally, and feel the leg muscles on the back of the thigh (hamstrings) gradually release their tension. This is a *static* stretch, because you are simply holding the position.

To add CR stretching to this exercise, keep your hands still, and press your leg downwards (hip extension) against the resistance of your hands. Your leg pushes down and your hands pull up, so nothing actually moves (an isometric contraction), but your hamstring muscles over the back of your thigh tense. Hold this muscle tension for five seconds and then release the tension, allowing your leg to lower slightly. Have a breather for 5–10 seconds, and then perform the static stretch again (pulling your leg up using only your hands, but keeping the leg muscles relaxed). You should now see that you can lift your leg slightly higher, and the feeling in your leg changes. Usually the sharp, slightly painful sensation of the stretch becomes dull and more pleasant. It's a little like taking a kettle off the boil!

Generally, to convert a static stretch into a CR stretch, simply tighten the muscles you are going to stretch, while trying to pull in the opposite direction, but without actually allowing movement. To take another example, your calf muscles are stretched by adopting a lunge position where your toes are pulled *upwards* towards your body. To perform CR, you use a toe-pointing action, pulling your toes *downwards* before you stretch

---

 KEY POINT

Contract–relax (CR) stretching is intense and can be used to increase the effectiveness of static stretching. To perform CR, first tense the muscle in the opposite direction from the stretching action.

What to expect from stretching

If you use intensive stretching, either by stretching quite far into your range, or by holding the stretch for longer than about 5–10 seconds, you may find that you are quite sore the next day. Even if you use a fairly brief programme, if it is very intensive you may be as sore as if you had played an intensive game.

There are two reasons for this. Soreness immediately after exercise is due to the build-up of naturally occurring acids within the working muscles. Soreness a day or two after exercise is called *delayed onset muscle soreness*, or DOMS for short. This occurs quite naturally during very intense exercise due to minor swelling around the fibres within the stretched muscle. It is quite harmless, but you should not stretch while your muscles are still sore in this way. Instead, use a warm bath and gentle massage to reduce the soreness.

Muscle soreness can also be reduced by using a cool-down after your workout. This should include similar exercises to those you used in your warm-up. The idea is to flush fresh blood through the muscles which have been worked to get rid of the acids which have been building up as you exercise.

Intense stretching is not recommended before playing a game, as it is likely to result in reduced output from the muscles. CR stretching should be an entirely separate part of your training programme.

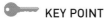 **KEY POINT**

Use a cool-down after exercise to reduce muscle soreness.

Some forms of exercise can give you quite rapid progress. For example, if you weight-train, you can often feel your muscles begin to tone relatively quickly – even within a few weeks. With stretching, however, progress is somewhat slower. It can take two to three months to begin to notice a change, although sometimes progress may be faster. One of the things we aim to do with stretching is to enable a tight muscle to relax. For example, you might have tight, sore shoulder muscles from sitting at a desk all day. When you stretch, you will notice the soreness go quite quickly, but the muscle will not actually lengthen for some months.

Even though progress in stretching can be slow, you will

22

notice that it is fairly continuous. If you join a yoga class, for example, you will notice that you continue to improve for some years after you begin. There are obviously physical limitations to progress – if you are 60, no amount of stretching will make you 16 again. However, many people in their sixties find themselves a lot more flexible than they were in their thirties and forties, simply because at the time – often when their children were growing up, and they led busy lives – they did not allow themselves time to exercise and so got into poor physical condition. Now they have time to train and they see progress.

3

Exercises

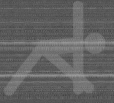

	Exercise	Static	Dynamic	Can CR be added?
	Phase I			
I.1	Hamstrings – active knee extension	✔	✘	✔
I.2	Rectus femoris stretch – standing	✔	✘	✔
I.3	Calf lunge	✔	✘	✔
I.4	Thoracic spine – kneeling	✔	✘	✘
I.5	Spinal rotation – lying	✔	✘	✔
I.6	Hip flexors / extensors – modified lunge	✔	✘	✘
	Phase II			
II.1	Anterior chest and shoulders	✔	✘	✔
II.2	Lateral flexion – standing	✔	✘	✔
II.3	Anterior tibials	✔	✘	✘
II.4	Hip adductors – long sit-	✔	✘	✘
II.5	ting Knee extension – with	✔	✘	✔
II.6	towel	✔	✘	✔
II.7	Hip flexors – Thomas test	✔	✘	✘
II.8	Deep calf and Achilles Wrist extensors – against	✔	✘	✘
	a wall			
III.1	*Phase III* Hip adductors –	✔	✘ ✔	✔
III.2	wall support	✔	✘	✘
III.3	Gluteals	✔	✘	✔
III.4	Hip flexors – supine lying	✔	✘	✔
III.5	Hamstring – lying on back Leg swing forwards and	✘	✔	✘
III.6	backwards	✘	✔	✘
III.7	Leg swing – sideways	✔	✘ ✔	✔
III.8	Calf stretch – sprint start Shoulder rotation with	✔	✘	✘
	towel			
III.9	Lying backwards	✔	✘ ✔	✔

3. Exercises

Phase I: Beginner

Phase I is the beginning phase. This does not mean you are a beginner to racquet sports, but simply that you are stretching in this way for the first time.

In this phase we are targeting the muscles used in racquet sports, but also using two exercises to loosen the spine. This is important, because all racquet sports pull unequally on one side of the body (they are asymmetrical), meaning that one side will be tighter and stronger than the other. As you perform the stretches, try to pull a little further into the tight side to redress this imbalance. This will even up your posture and make sure your spine moves an equal amount in both directions.

This phase lays the foundation for the next two phases, using slightly simpler exercises that are nevertheless very effective. As all the stretches in phase I are static, begin by holding each movement for three to five seconds. Make sure you don't hold your breath, but instead focus your attention on breathing out, as you will often notice that your muscles relax during this time. You can expect your muscles to feel comfortably sore as you stretch, but not painful. If you are very inflexible and the exercises are painful, keep the holding time the same, but release the stretch slightly so that you are pushing just to the beginning of the feeling of stiffness but not right into it. Perform a maximum of two repetitions for each movement. Generally you can perform all the phase I exercises in a single daily session, but if you are short of time you can perform half in the morning and half in the afternoon. However, remember to do a warm-up before both sessions!

If you were to measure your discomfort on a scale of 1 to 10, with 1 being no discomfort and 10 being very painful indeed, your stretching at the beginning of phase I should only measure 2–3 on the comfort scale.

During the second week you can stretch further into your stiffness range, but even so your discomfort should never be greater than 5 on the scale. Increase the number of reps to three or four, and hold each for 6–10 seconds. During week three try to hold each rep for 20–30 seconds, and perform five reps. As a guide, a 20–30 second hold corresponds to about five complete breaths (in and out)! This is quite intense stretching now, so it may feel uncomfortable, perhaps 6–7 on the comfort scale. Because you may be sore following this training, perform the exercises on alternate days to allow adequate recovery. You may actually need longer than this to recover. The best guide is not to begin a stretching exercise if the muscles to be stretched are still very sore (above 5 on the comfort scale) from the last session.

Although there are only six exercises in this section, you may find it too time-consuming to perform five reps of each in every training session as recommended for week three. Don't drop any of the exercises, however, as this will leave certain muscles unstretched and risk muscle imbalance. Instead, limit yourself to two well-performed reps, holding the first for 20 seconds, and the second for 30.

KEY POINT

Racquet sports use your muscles unevenly (asymmetrically). Use your new stretching programme to correct unequal muscle tightness which may have developed over the years.

SUMMARY – TRAINING IN PHASE I

Week 1
- Hold for 3–5 seconds
- Mild discomfort only
- Two reps per training session
- Daily practice

Week 2
- Hold for 6–10 seconds
- Slight muscle burning
- Three to four reps per training session
- Daily practice

Week 3
- Hold for 20–30 seconds
- Tolerable muscle burning, but NOT PAIN
- Five reps maximum for each exercise
- Alternate days

Note
Where exercises are described on one side of the body (for example the right leg) you should perform the same exercise on the other side (left leg).

I.1 Hamstrings – active knee extension

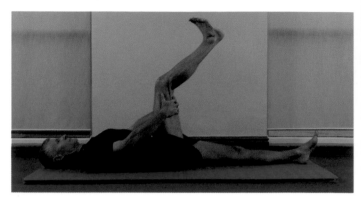

Lie with your back on the floor with your left leg straight and bend your right knee and hip to 90 degrees. Grip your hands behind the right knee and straighten your leg using the power of your quadriceps (the muscle in the front of the thigh) alone. The knee should remain directly above the hip – don't allow it to fall downwards, and your toes should remain relaxed. Rest for 10 seconds before repeating.

Variations

Place your hand on the front of your leg and actively push the leg on to your hand using the power of your hip muscles; at the same time, extend your knee. This will cause the hamstring muscles (on the back of the leg) to relax further through a natural reflex action. This technique can be useful if your hamstrings are very tight, or if they have a tendency to cramp and go into spasm.

Points to note

• Pulling your toes towards you and flexing your neck will throw stress on to the delicate sciatic nerve running along the back of your leg, and away from the hamstrings. This is a useful procedure in some cases, but is best performed under the supervision of a physiotherapist.

I.2 Rectus femoris stretch

Stand side-on to a wall with your right hand supporting your body-weight. Bend your left leg and grip your ankle keeping your knee bent. Pull your left hip back into back (extension), while maintaining correct spinal alignment.

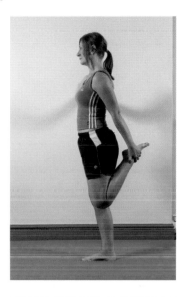

Loop a towel around your ankle to reduce the amount of knee bend and allow you to pull your hip further back. This will emphasise the upper portion of the muscle.

If this becomes a favourite exercise, you can use it in phases II and III as a CR technique. At the point of maximum stretch, try to straighten your leg at the same time, holding your ankle firmly. Nothing will move, but your rectus femoris muscle will tighten (isometric contraction) and as you release you should find that you can stretch a little further.

Points to note

- The rectus femoris is one of the quadriceps muscles, and acts to extend the leg at the knee. The exercise also stretches the femoral nerve at the front of the thigh.
- A sensation of burning or tingling (pins and needles) over the front of the thigh suggests that this nerve may be tight or possibly trapped, requiring management with physiotherapy.

I.3 Calf lunge

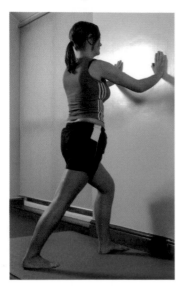

Begin by facing a wall in a half-lunge position with your left foot forward. Place your hands on the wall and bend your arms to lower your body forwards, encouraging your left foot to bend upwards (dorsiflexion).

Variations

Altering the angle of the foot away from the perpendicular will change the emphasis on the calf muscle. Pressing the knee over the outside of the foot will stretch the inner calf. Pressing it over the inside of the foot will stretch the outer calf.

Points to note

- Your heel must remain on the floor throughout the movement.
- As the knee is straight in this movement, the stretch on the superficial calf muscle (gastrocnemius) is increased and that on the deep calf muscle (soleus) reduced.

I.4 Thoracic spine – kneeling

Kneeling on all fours, sit back on your ankles, keeping your hands fixed. You should feel the stretch in the muscles at the sides of your upper body (latissimus dorsi).

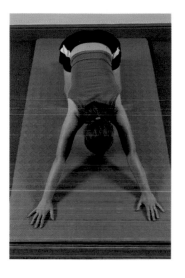

33

I.5 Spinal rotation – lying

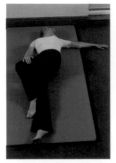 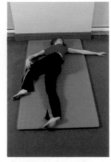

Lie on your back on the floor with your left arm out at 90 degrees. Bend your left knee and twist your trunk towards the right leg, bringing your left knee towards the floor. You will feel the stretch both on your back and the outside of your hip.

Variations

You can take the stretch further by gently pressing on your right knee to encourage (but not force) it towards the ground. This type of action is called 'overpressure'.

If you find the stretch too difficult, place a cushion on the floor and take your knee down onto the cushion. Alternatively, adjusting the degree of bend at your hip and knee will alter the stress of the stretch.

If you have spasms in your back muscles throughout the day, converting this exercise to a CR stretch may help. As you press down on your right knee with your hand, twist your trunk and press your left leg upwards against your hand. Your hand and knee press with equal and opposite force so nothing actually moves. Hold this tension for five seconds and then release, allowing the knee to lower further towards the ground.

Points to note

Because this action involves leverage, it should be performed in a slow and controlled manner. As the rotation occurs, the lower hip will tuck under the body. This is fine, as it becomes the pivot point around which your body moves.

I.6 Hip flexors and extensors – modified lunge

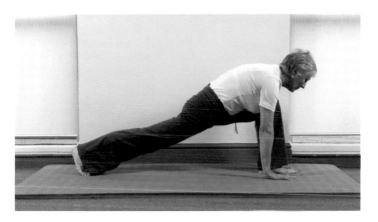

Start with your feet shoulder width apart. Step forwards with your left leg and lower your body towards the ground, supporting your weight with your hands. Keep your left foot flat and your knee and foot in line. You should feel the stretch in two places – on the buttock of the bent (left) leg and the top of the thigh of the straight (right) leg.

Variations
Placing the hands on the inside of the bent leg rather than the outside will increase the stretch.

Points to note
Because your full body weight is being used, you must perform this exercise slowly.

Phase II: Intermediate

The exercises in this phase will stretch a greater variety of muscles, including those used directly in racquet sports such as the front of the legs (quadriceps), back of the legs (hamstrings), inside and outside of the thigh (adductors and abductors) and calf muscles. They also address areas where tightness builds up in the lower back and shoulders.

The exercises build on the foundations laid in phase I, and although we are using new exercises, it is fine to swap in any exercises from phase I that you found of particular benefit for your body.

Begin as before by holding each movement for three to five seconds, focusing on breathing out to help your muscles to relax. You only need to perform a maximum of two repetitions for each movement. As with phase I, pay attention to your discomfort levels. In phase I you did not exceed a score of 2–3 on your comfort scale (10 being the worst possible pain), and in phase II you should aim to score the same or slightly higher, perhaps up to 4, but no more. Discomfort is to be expected with intense training, but real pain normally means you have pushed yourself too far and are likely to be injured.

For the second week stretch further into your stiffness range once more, and increase the number of reps to three or four, with a hold of 6–10 seconds. Finally, in week three, try to hold each rep for 20–30 seconds, performing five reps. As with phase I, in weeks one and two you can perform the exercises daily. In week 3 you may again be quite sore, so stretch on alternate days.

There is no need to perform all the exercises in each session. There are eight exercises in phase II, so try to pick three or four per day so that you have used all eight every two or three days. Splitting the programme up in this way (a method known as periodisation) allows your muscles time to recover. Your aim should be never to use intense stretching on a muscle which is still sore from a previous training bout.

SUMMARY – TRAINING IN PHASE II
Week 1
- Hold for 3–5 seconds
- Moderate discomfort only
- Two reps
- Daily training
- Continue to use any phase I exercises you found especially beneficial

Week 2
- Hold for 6–10 seconds
- Slight muscle burning
- Three to four reps
- Daily training

Week 3
- Hold for 20–30 seconds
- Slight muscle burning
- Five reps
- Alternate days.

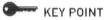 **KEY POINT**

Do not use intense stretching on a muscle which is still sore from a previous training session.

II.1 Anterior chest and shoulders

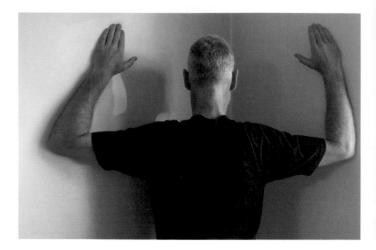

Stand facing a doorway or the corner of a room with your upper arms out to your sides at shoulder level and elbows bent to 90 degrees. Lean forwards, pressing your chest through the doorway or into the corner, forcing your arms back into extension. You should feel the stretch over the front of your chest.

Variations

Increasing and reducing the height of your arms will vary the focus of the stretch.

Points to note

Because the full body weight is being supported by your upper body, heavy individuals and those with poor shoulder flexibility should take up a lunge position, moving some of the body weight on to the front foot.

II.2 Lateral flexion – standing

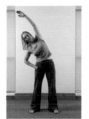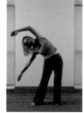

Stand with your feet shoulder width apart. Bend your spine sideways (side flexion), placing your right arm on your waist or thigh to support your body weight. Take your left arm above your head to increase the stretch.

This movement stretches the side bending muscles on the upper (left) side of the body.

Variations

Place both arms on your waist to reduce the overload. Stretching both hands overhead increases the overload on the spine, and changes the emphasis of the exercise from stretch to strength.

Points to note

- Asymmetry in the side bending action of the spine is common in racquet sports, so you may find that your degree of movement is greater on one side than the other.
- The photograph on the left shows the exercise being performed correctly: the subject's right hand is on her hip, taking the weight of her trunk, and the curve of her spine is gentle. The right-hand photo is incorrect, because the subject has not placed her hand on her waist for support. As her whole upper bodyweight is now pressing down on the spine, she has bent further but the curve of her spine is no longer gentle. In addition, because her body is forced further down her left hip is now pressed sideways and she no longer takes her weight equally over both feet – her posture is less stable and she could easily topple over.

II.3 Anterior tibials

Kneel on the floor and then sit back on your ankles, pressing the front of the ankles to the floor. You should feel the stretch along the outside of your shin bone (anterior tibial muscles).

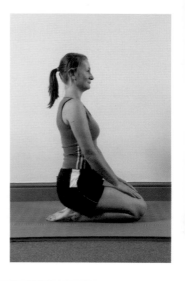

Variations

Place a folded towel beneath your toes to press them into flexion and increase the stretch on the toe extensor muscles.

Points to note

- This exercise can place considerable stress on your knees. If you experience knee pain, perform the exercise leaning on a stool to support your body weight.
- If you have ever suffered from a broken ankle, you may not be able to perform this exercise. You will feel the stretch on your stiff ankle rather than on your shin muscles. See a physiotherapist to determine which ankle stretching exercises are appropriate for your condition.

II.4 Hip adductors – long sitting

Sit on the floor with both legs
straight. Bend your right leg,
placing your foot on your left thigh
above the knee. Support your foot
with your left hand, and press
down on your right knee with your
right hand. You should feel the
stretch on the inside of your thigh,
travelling up into the groin.
Lengthen your spine and maintain
good spinal alignment throughout
the movement.

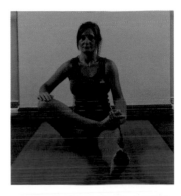

Variations

Start by sitting with your back
flat against a wall with a rolled
towel placed in the small of your
back (lumbar area) to maintain
spinal alignment. You can also
sit on a wedge to tip your pelvis

forwards. If your knee is too stiff
to bend enough to allow your
foot to rest on your thigh, rest
your foot on the shin just below
your knee instead.

Points to note

- Most individuals are
asymmetrical and will find
that one leg is more flexible
than the other.
- Those who have reduced
flexibility of the muscles on the
inside of the thigh may have a
tendency to tilt the body
towards the bent knee, lifting
the pelvis and buttock from the
floor. This gives an apparent
increase in flexibility as the

knee can be lowered further,
but in fact does not create any
more stretch in these muscles.
- Do not perform this exercise
(except under the supervision
of a physiotherapist) if you
have suffered from Pubic
Symphasis Dysfunction (PSD)
after recent childbirth.

II.5 Knee extension – with towel

Lie with your back on the floor with your left leg straight, and bend your right knee and hip to an angle of 90 degrees from the floor. Hook a folded towel around your right foot, holding one end of the towel in each hand. Now try to straighten your leg by pushing your foot into the towel. Do not allow your arms to straighten, and keep the hip, knee and foot in a straight line.

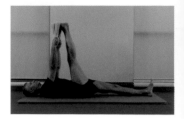

Variations

Instead of a towel, use an exercise band. Make sure that the band is in the centre of the foot rather than around the toes to prevent it from slipping.

Points to note

- Fastening the towel over your toes will pull the toes towards you.
- Combining this movement with bending (flexion) of the neck will throw stress on to the nerves and away from the hamstring muscles. This is a technique often used by physiotherapists to stretch a tight nerve after injury. Although useful, you should not continue the stretch if you get pins and needles in your leg, as this means too much stress is being placed on the nerve.

II.6 Hip flexors – Thomas test position

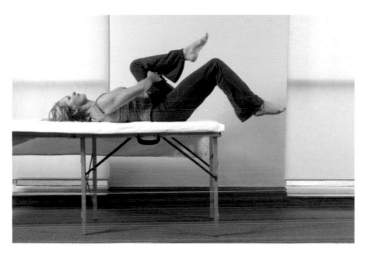

Lie with your back on a bench or stable dining table and your right leg over the bench ond. Bend your left hip and knee and pull your knee towards your chest. You will feel the stretch on the lower leg, along the front of the thigh and up into the front of the hip.

Variations

Start with both knees bent and the feet flat on the bench. Pull one knee to the chest and then lower the opposite leg.

Points to note

* This movement is known as the Thomas test, a test used in physiotherapy to assess hip flexor muscle tightness.

II.7 Deep calf and Achilles

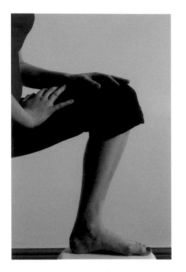

Place a low stool or chair against a wall to stop it sliding. Put your left foot in the centre of the chair, place your right foot on the floor and slightly to the side of the chair, and take up a lunge position. Keeping your foot flat, and your heel in contact with the chair seat, press your knee forwards over your toes.

Variations

Altering the angle of the foot away from the perpendicular will change the emphasis on the deep calf and Achilles.

By bending the knee, the emphasis is taken away from the long superficial calf muscle (gastrocnemius) and placed on the shorter, deep calf muscles (soleus and tibialis posterior). This is a useful alternative to try once each week for variety.

Points to note

- Your heel must remain on the chair seat throughout the movement. Raising the heel takes the emphasis away from the deep calf and Achilles and throws it onto the foot itself.

II.8 Wrist extensors – against a wall

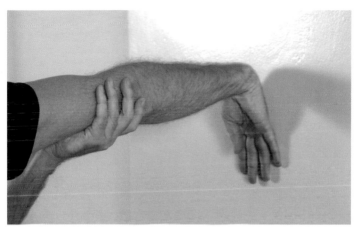

Stand facing a wall about an arm's length away from it. Place the back of your right hand flat on the wall with your fingers vertical and straighten your arm. Use your left hand to lock your right elbow and maintain the locked position throughout the movement. Lean forwards towards the wall, pressing your wrist into further flexion.

Variations

Placing your hand higher up the wall will increase the range of motion.

Points to note

- Where you feel an ache close to the elbow, the muscle is being stretched.
- When the sensation is over the wrist, the wrist extensor tendons on the back of the forearm are being stretched, rather than the full muscle. Unless this area is very tight, stick to the straight arm stretch

Phase III: Advanced

Phase III maintains the theme of the previous phases: the exercises here target both the muscles involved in racquet sports, and those body areas which tend to get stiff as a result of the racquet sports posture. As well as the spine, you will be stretching out the chest and shoulders, because this area tends to tighten if you develop a round-shouldered posture and can often give a burning pain between the shoulder blades.

In addition to the static stretches seen in phases I and II, we introduce dynamic stretches to prepare you for the rapid stretching needed during the more explosive sequences of a game.

In this phase we perform the programme with the same repetitions and holding times as phases I and II. However, the phase III movements are generally more challenging, so make sure you really focus on good exercise technique. Make sure you don't bounce into the movements or hold your breath. Be sure to follow the exercise instructions closely and be aware of your body alignment. In phases I and II we took three weeks to complete the whole phase. For phase III, you may use this weekly timing as a guide, but it is best to progress only when you are ready.

Begin holding each movement for three to five seconds, and perform two reps of each movement. Progress to three or four reps, with a hold for 6–10 seconds, when you feel ready. Select the exercises which you find most beneficial and perform these, holding each rep for 20–30 seconds and performing five reps.

How will you know when you are ready to move on? Remember that you must not stretch if you are still sore from the day before. If you are not sore, try to hold the movement for longer (except for exercises III.5 and III.6 which are dynamic stretches). If you are able to hold the movement correctly without wobbling or feeling that it is very painful (8 on the comfort scale) you can move on.

There are nine exercises in phase III, so pick three or four per day and you will use all of them every two to three days.

You may now consider increasing the intensity of your stretching by adding some contract–relax (CR) movements after you have performed two reps of your static stretching. The exercise descriptions explain how to do this.

SUMMARY – TRAINING IN PHASE III

To begin:
- Hold for 3–5 seconds
- Moderate discomfort only
- Two reps

Progress when ready to:
- Holding for 6–10 seconds
- Slight muscle burning
- Three to four reps

Progress when ready to:
- Holding for 20–30 seconds
- Slight muscle burning
- Five reps
- Consider using CR stretching where appropriate.

🔑 **KEY POINT**

Phase III training is more intense, but make sure you keep each movement under control.

III.1 Hip adductors – wall support

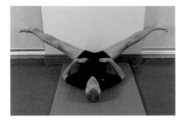

Lie with your back on the floor with your legs straight up in the air and your buttocks close to a wall. Rest your legs against the wall and allow them to lower slowly out to the sides and downwards (this is known as hip adduction). You should feel the stretch on the inside of the thigh right up into the groin. Hold this position (static stretch) for 20–30 seconds and then bring your legs back up again by 20–30 cm (resisted adduction), before again allowing them to lower.

Variations

Lifting the legs against their own weight provides resistance for contract–relax (CR) stretching. This resistance can be increased by having a training partner resist the adduction movement for you by pressing down on your legs.

If you perform this action rhythmically – one rep per complete movement – the action becomes a dynamic stretch. In this case, you do not hold the fully stretched position (legs in the lower position) but instead lift the legs up again straight away. This is a useful variation to put in perhaps once each week.

Points to note

- Although this is obviously a stretching exercise, because the legs are lifted against their own weight you will also gain adductor muscle strength.

III.2 Gluteals

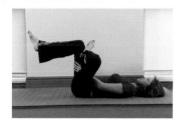

Lie with your back on the floor. Bend your left leg at the hip and knee – about 90° angle at each. Then draw your right knee up, pressing it on to your left foot. Reach around your right knee or thigh and pull your knee towards your right shoulder, pressing your left hip into an outward twisting position (external rotation). You should feel the stretch in your buttock and on the outside of your right hip.

Variations

Altering the position of your left leg (either by twisting it more or less or pulling it up more or less) will change the emphasis of the stretch. Alter the leg position so that you feel most comfortable when holding the stretch.

Points to note

- This exercise also places stress on the pelvis, so it should not be used for three months after childbirth.
- If you are unable to bend your hip high enough to grip around your thigh, loop a towel around your thigh and grip that instead.

III.3 Hip flexors – supine lying (with partner)

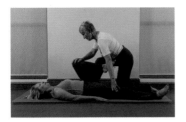

Lie on the floor on your back, with your left hip and knee bent. Your partner should half kneel at your left hip. With her left hand she holds your right leg on the floor, and with her right hand presses your left leg closer to your chest (hip flexion).

This movement stretches the hip flexor muscles of the lower leg, and the buttock of the upper leg.

Variations

If you experience pain in your flexed knee, your partner should place her hand on the underside of the knee, to avoid compressing the joint.

If you do not have a partner, you can perform the exercise yourself, simply pulling your own knee in to your chest. The advantage of having a partner do this for you, however, is that you are able to relax all your muscles as the stretch is put on.

Points to note

- Most individuals are asymmetrical, so one leg may appear less flexible than the other.
- Do not perform this stretch if you have had a hip joint replacement.

III.4 Hamstrings – lying on back (with partner)

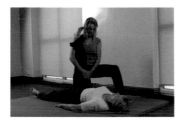

Lie on the floor on your back, with your legs straight. Your partner should half kneel at your right hip and lift your right leg, placing her hand over your right knee to keep the leg straight. With your leg resting on your partner's shoulder she should lunge forwards, pressing your leg further upwards (hip flexion). Hold this stretched position (static stretch) by trying to relax your leg on your partner's shoulder. Slowly release the stretch as your partner lowers your leg.

Variations

Place a small pad on your partner's shoulder and a small rolled towel under your back to make the position more comfortable.

To increase the stretch further, perform the exercise as a CR technique. With your partner holding your leg, press the leg downwards (hip extension) as your partner presses against you. Tense the muscles without any movement (isometric contraction) and as you relax, have your partner press your leg further upwards, performing the static stretch described above.

Points to note

• When locking your leg out straight, make sure that the pressure is not placed directly over your kneecap. Your partner should cup her hand and place it around, but not directly on top of, your knee.

51

III.5 Leg swing – forwards and backwards

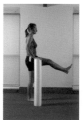 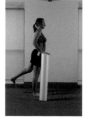

Stand with your feet shoulder width apart. Hold on to a bar or the frame of a piece of gym apparatus or furniture at your right side for balance. Swing your left leg forwards and upwards (hip flexion), first to shin level, then to waist level and eventually to chest level. You will feel the stretch on the back of your thigh (hamstring muscles) as your leg swings forwards, and on the front of the thigh (hip flexors) as it swings backwards.

Progress the range of motion as you feel comfortable, being careful not to overstretch. As your leg goes backwards, maintain your low back alignment – do not allow your back to hollow excessively.

Variations

Keeping the leg straight places the stretch on the hip. If you let the knee bend, as though kicking your backside, you will stretch the thigh muscles right down to your knee as well.

Points to note

- Ensure that the action is controlled throughout the whole movement range.
- Do not allow the momentum to pull you into a range that you would not normally use.
- Too much speed will force your pelvis to tip forwards, hollowing your back excessively.

III.6 Leg swing – sideways

Stand facing a piece of gym equipment or high cupboard with your feet hip width apart. Hold on to the apparatus with both hands. Shift your pelvis to the left to take your whole weight onto your left leg and unload your right. Swing your right leg out to the side and then inwards and in front of the left leg (abduction and adduction). Start by swinging outwards to shin level, then knee level and finally hip level. As you swing your leg, do not allow your trunk to twist.

As the leg swings outwards,

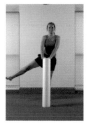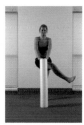

you will feel the stretch on the inside of your thigh up to your groin (adductor muscles) and as it swings inwards you will feel it over the outside of the hip and thigh (abductors).

Variations

Pointing your heel to the ceiling (toes to the floor) combines swinging outwards (abduction) with twisting inwards (medial rotation). Pointing your toes to the ceiling combines hip abduction with lateral rotation. Use both actions to balance your training programme unless your medial rotators are especially long, in which case the lateral rotation movement alone should be emphasised. With this variation, because the rotators of the hip are also targeted, you may also feel the stretch deep inside the hip joint itself.

Points to note

- In order to unload the swinging leg, you must transfer your body weight over the other (weight-bearing) leg. You can achieve this by shifting your pelvis over the weight-bearing leg.

- If you lack hip control and hip stability, you may find that you simply tip your spine sideways. Try to avoid this by keeping your spine upright and your pelvis level.

53

III.7 Calf stretch – sprint start

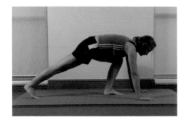

Stand in a lunge position with your right leg back and your left leg forwards, with your weight over your front leg. Place the toes of your back foot on the ground and gradually take your weight backwards, forcing your heel onto the ground as you do so. Pause, then use the calf strength of your back leg to 'flick' you forwards as though exploding out of the blocks from a sprint start. Repeat the exercise five times with the right leg back, then reverse the movement.

Variations

Placing your back leg further back will increase the intensity of the stretch; taking your leg further forwards will reduce it.

You can emphasise the power aspect of this movement rather than the stretch by taking more weight on to your back leg and jumping slightly as you flick yourself forwards. This then becomes a dynamic stretch. Use this if you have suffered from a calf injury after you have had physiotherapy treatment and used static stretching for four to six weeks. Before you play again, the dynamic stretch will prepare you for explosive actions in sport such as lunging for a deep ball.

Points to note

- Make sure you build the range of motion progressively. Start with your feet quite close together and gradually move your back leg further backwards as your confidence in the movement grows.

III.8 Combined shoulder rotation with towel

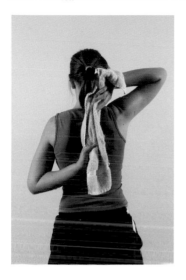

Grasp a towel behind your back with your right arm placed behind your neck and your left arm in the small of your back. Move your arms up and down to lift and lower the towel vertically.

Variations

A broom handle or your racquet can be used instead of the towel, or, if you are very flexible, you may be able to grasp your hands together. If you perform the exercise sitting or kneeling on the floor, bending the trunk slightly forwards will increase the intensity of the stretch by pressing the lower arm further backwards.

Points to note

- Asymmetry in shoulder rotation is common, so the range of motion may differ when you swap your arm positions.

III.9 Lying backward trunk twist

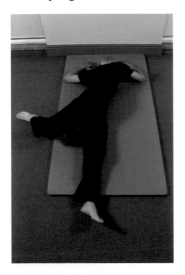

Lie on your front on a mat. Reach your arms out in front of you, keeping your elbows comfortably bent. Your chest and head should be flat on the floor. Lift your right leg and take it upwards and backwards across your left leg. As you do this, allow your trunk to bend backwards and twist, opening up your ribcage on the right hand side. Reverse the movement on the left side of the body.

You will feel the stretch over the right side of the body, in the small of your back and over the thigh of your right leg. There is also some stretch on your shoulders.

Variations

Bend your leg more to increase the stretch on the front thigh muscles (quadriceps) and less to reduce the stretch over the spine.

This is a static stretch, held at the end of the movement. You can make this stretch dynamic by lowering the leg and then lifting it back to the starting position without a rest. Make sure you keep the movement slow and controlled, however – a fast drop of the leg will place excessive stress on the lower back.

Points to note

• Make sure you feel an even stretch on the trunk and hip. If you have very stiff hips, you will find that your spine will compensate and stretch further. To avoid this, place a cushion on the floor on the left side of your body so your foot can rest on the cushion at the point of maximum stretch. This will release some of the stretch on the hip and spine.

Maintaining your flexibility

When you have completed all three phases of the programme, you will have built up to intense stretching over about a nine- or ten-week period. You now have a choice – to maintain your current stretching level, or to continue to develop further flexibility on problem areas. If you found any of the exercises really hard, and were not able to stretch to the degree you would like, continue with these movements. Practise these at the beginning of your stretching workout when you are fresh.

To maintain your new-found level of flexibility, pick three exercises from the programme and practise daily, changing the three you select each day. Rest from stretching for either one day per week or two if you find you are very sore. In this way you will be using a total of 15 or 18 different stretching exercises each week and maintaining your level of flexibility with a good variety of movements.

If you find this too demanding, you should try to stretch at least three times per week, using the following exercises.

- Exercise I.1: hamstrings – active knee extension
- Exercise I.2: rectus femoris stretch – standing
- Exercise II.7: deep calf and Achilles
- Exercise III.1: hip adductors wall support.

Use alternate days (Monday, Wednesday, Friday, for example) and practise each of the exercises in a single session. As part of pre-game preparation you can use these stretches following a general warm-up. In this case, use static stretching, holding each stretch for three to five seconds, and perform each movement twice. If you are stretching on a day when you will not play, you can increase the holding to 20–30 seconds and perform four or five reps of each exercise.

4

When things go wrong

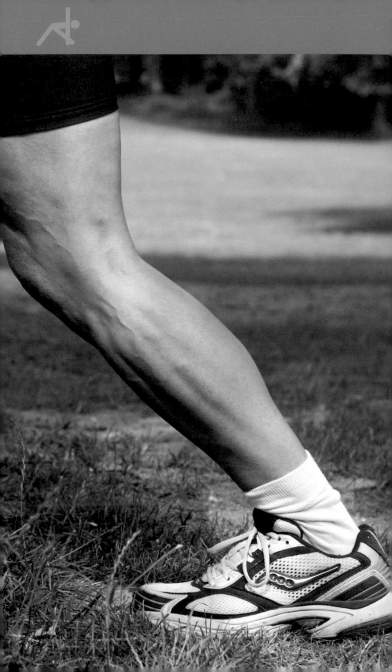

4. When things go wrong

However careful you are with your training or competition, at some time you are likely to be injured. Injuries normally occur in one of two ways.

A sudden (or *traumatic*) injury occurs when you trip or fall, or when you twist suddenly and feel something 'go'. This is more usual when you are tired towards the end of a game, and as a consequence become less coordinated. It may also happen when you do too much too soon, rather than building up your training gradually. Either way, the effect on the body is the same – the injured tissues bleed and swell internally. If the injury is bad, this may be seen on the surface of the body as bruising and swelling.

The second type of injury is almost the reverse. In this type, injury comes on gradually, and often unnoticed – a so-called *overuse* condition. Overuse may occur if your training is too intense and you have not allowed your body enough time between sessions to recover. Another factor can be a body alignment fault, where one part of your body keeps taking excessive strain, rather than allowing stress to be shared evenly over several body areas. Typical alignment faults in racquet sports include foot problems, such as excessive pronation (flatfooted posture), and poor shoulder alignment as a result of faulty technique when striking the ball overhead.

In both injury types, your initial course of action should be rest. In the case of trauma, you can use cold or ice to slow down the injury process, and with overuse you need to look closely at your training to see if there are any technique faults.

Home first aid for sports injury

So, you were playing your final set, lunged for a wide shot, lost your footing and twisted your ankle. You hobbled off court; you have driven home and taken your trainers off. What should you do now – have a hot bath? Rub in some cream? Use some strapping? Apply some ice? The answer is RICE:

- Rest
- Ice

61

- Compression
- Elevation.

Let's use the ankle as an example of correct injury management, although the actions below are the same for any injury.

Rest
Initially you should rest, rather than try to work the injury off. Try to keep your foot up (see below) and if you do have to walk, use crutches or a stick if you can, to avoid putting stress on the healing tissues.

Ice
Use ice or a cold pack. There are many commercially available types. Some contain granules and a fluid which you squeeze to mix the chemicals, so making the pack cold. Others are gel packs which you keep in the fridge. If you don't have either of these, just use a packet of frozen peas from the freezer. They will do just as well, and will mould around the injury.

Before you start, however, remember never to put an ice pack directly in contact with your skin – it will cause an ice burn which is very painful. Instead, wrap the pack in a damp tea towel, which will protect the skin but still conduct the cold into the tissues. Keep the pack on for 10–20 minutes, and re-apply it two or three times a day for the next three days.

During this three day period, swelling is still forming. After this, probably no fresh swelling will develop, so although your ankle stills appears swollen, it is old swelling rather than new. Once the swelling has stopped forming, you can stop using the ice.

 KEY POINT
Never put an ice pack directly onto the skin, as it can cause a painful burn. Wrap the pack in a wet cloth or tea towel first.

Compression

Swelling is caused by a sticky fluid, which if unchecked will spread over the tissues near the injury and stick them together, making the area stiff. To prevent this, use compression. The simplest method is an elastic tubular bandage from a chemist. If you don't have one, wrap a standard crepe bandage around the ankle. Failing this, use a tea towel instead. The compression should be comfortable: if you feel your ankle throbbing, it is probably too tight, so remove it and re-apply it slightly less tightly.

Elevation

With lower limb injuries (those to the ankle, knee or hip) the watery swelling tends to be pulled down by gravity and form a thick pool around your ankle bones. To prevent this, rest with your leg up or elevated on a stool. Raise it at least to the horizontal or slightly above. This will make your return to sport far quicker.

Elevate your leg for three days after injury, while swelling is forming. Later, if you find your leg has a tendency to swell if you do too much on it, you can still use elevation to reduce the swelling at any time. If the swelling is stubborn a good trick is to put a cushion between your mattress and bed base at night. This will provide a few inches of elevation, which is not enough to stop you sleeping, but just enough to reduce the swelling overnight.

Getting back into sport

Once the pain and swelling begin to ease (about three to five days after injury) you can begin very gentle exercise to help loosen the stiff tissues. The trick is to get a balance between doing just enough to ease the stiffness, but not too much so that you disrupt the healing tissues. The guide here is pain. If you begin with pain and it gradually eases, the chances are that you are simply easing off some stiffness. However, if the pain begins to increase, you should stop, as it means you are doing too much and the tissues will start to swell again. The golden rule of rehabilitation (exercise following injury) is never to exercise through increasing pain.

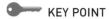

> 🔑 **KEY POINT**
> Never exercise through increasing pain.

Begin with simple, non-weight-bearing movements, that is without taking your weight through the injury. In the case of the ankle, for example, gently circle the ankle and flex it up and down. For a knee, sit on a table or stool and slowly bend and straighten your knee. As you feel the movement tightening, gradually try to ease into the stiff region. If the movement slowly begins to increase, that's fine – you can continue for 5–10 reps and then rest. Have a breather and then start again, aiming to perform two sets of 10 reps twice each day.

About one or two weeks after the injury you will be ready to use stretching exercises. Remember the golden rule not to work through increasing pain. Remember also that stretching, although the topic of this book, is not the only fitness component you should work on during a rehabilitation programme. You will need to re-strengthen your injured limb and also build up the muscle endurance. An important factor following any injury is stability of the limb – how capable your muscles are of supporting your joint and holding it firm. This, combined with exercises to develop the sense of balance in the limb, is often the final deciding factor between getting back into sport and suffering setbacks.

It is always best to perform your rehabilitation under the guidance of a qualified physiotherapist. An expert will often see things about your injury that you cannot, so a visit to your physio is a good investment.

Let's have a look now at some specific injuries seen in racquet sports and the best stretching exercises to use to aid recovery.

Sprained ankle

When you sprain your ankle, you are most likely to injure the ligament on the outside of the joint. This structure supports your ankle when it points in and down, and following injury it is often this movement which is tight and so needs to be stretched again.

The easiest way to stretch this area is to cross your injured leg at the shin over the uninjured one. Use one hand to steady the lower leg on the injured side, and cup the other around the foot and ankle to pull it down, round and inwards. The stretch should be gentle and held for 5–10 seconds, providing this does not increase the pain.

Once you have managed this, the next stage is to stretch your ankle actively by standing and rocking over on to the outer edge of your foot, or by walking on a slope. This movement is still slow and controlled, but eventually you can use faster actions to develop agility (stretch, balance and strength combined) in the ankle structures. One of the best ways to achieve an agile ankle joint is to walk on an uneven surface such as soft ground or sand. You can also make your own uneven surface by placing four or five cushions on the ground and walking, then slowly jogging, over them in bare feet. At each stage, the action must be controlled, so you don't feel that the movement is 'running away' with you.

As well as stretching the side of the ankle, walking on an uneven surface also strengthens the muscles surrounding the ankle so that they can support or stabilise the joint. Ankle stability is the most important aspect of fitness to develop following an ankle injury. You can also try this exercise:

- stand on one leg (the injured one) and hold this position for 20–30 seconds. When you do this, you will notice all the muscles around the ankle 'flickering' as they work hard to support the joint and hold it stable.
- Progress to standing on one leg and performing some show movements with your racquet.
- Finally try hitting the ball repeatedly while standing on one leg.

This last point may seem strange, but by focusing your attention on the ball, you are taking it away from the ankle and this in turn makes the work of the ankle muscle (which is stabilising the joint) more automatic – something which is vital when you are on court.

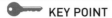

🔑 **KEY POINT**
Following a sprained ankle, stretch the outside of the joint
and stabilise it using single-leg standing actions.

Shin splints

Shin splints is a condition affecting the shin muscles
themselves. These are long muscles running alongside the two
shin bones (the tibia and fibula). The muscles are sandwiched
between the tight skin of your shin and the flat shin bones. With
training, the muscles swell and thicken and, as this happens,
they are unable to expand fully because of their sandwiched
position. Instead of expanding, pressure within them increases,
which cuts off their own blood supply. This reduction in blood
flow, combined with a build-up of acids within the muscles, gives
rise to the characteristic gnawing pain of shin splints.

Stretching exercises can help some types of shin splints by
preventing the muscles from becoming short and tight in the first
place.

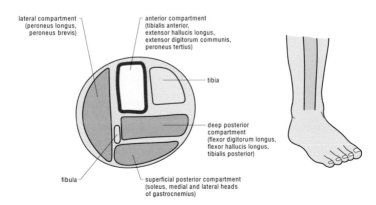

Compartments of the lower leg

On the front of the shin lie two sets of muscles, the anterior tibials and the toe extensors. These muscles pull the foot and toes upwards, an action used repeatedly as you play. To stretch these muscles, immediately after playing or training, you need to press the foot slowly downwards in the opposite direction, using exercise II.3. Hold the stretch (using a folded towel) for 30–60 seconds to allow the muscles to 'give' gradually. Repeat the stretch four or five times.

Pulled hamstring

When you tear a hamstring, you may injure the muscle in its centre part (called the belly) or at the end of the muscle (called the muscle-tendon or MT junction). The difference between these two areas is that the MT junction does not contract, while the muscle belly does. As well as stretching, muscle-belly tears will therefore need strength training to broaden the

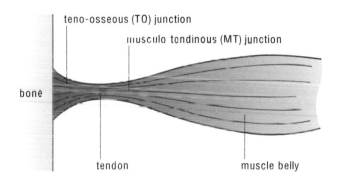

Areas of injury in a muscle

muscle and separate the individual muscle fibres to prevent them from sticking together. Injury to the MT junction often responds to stretching alone.

Because the hamstring muscles are involved in so many movements on court, you will need to use two types of stretches – static to regain the movement range, and dynamic to build up the 'whipping' action of the muscle, used as you lunge for a ball.

Use exercise I.1 to begin. Once this is comfortable, progress to the long sitting exercise shown here. You may use both exercises to begin with, but when you stretch for a longer period (20–30 second hold) use only the second exercise.

Hamstring stretch – long sitting exercise

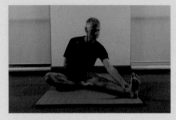 Sit with your injured leg straight and your other leg comfortably bent. Reach forwards with your hand on the side of the straight leg to grip the sole of your foot. Press the other hand on your straightened knee to maintain knee extension. Make sure you maintain spinal alignment by gently curving through the spine.

Ease into the movement, gradually increasing your movement range. Hold the comfortably stretched position initially for 10–15 seconds and then for 20–30 seconds; perform four or five reps. You should also perform some of the stretches with the knee slightly unlocked (bent). This will take the stretch away from the lower hamstrings and you will feel the stretch more focused on the upper muscle portion towards your buttock.

To redevelop the muscle's 'whipping' action, use the dynamic leg swinging exercise (III.5). Swing your leg initially to shin level and then to waist and finally chest height. Begin slowly and gradually build up speed. Once you are confident with this single direction movement (up and down), change to a multi-direction movement, kicking across the body (up, down and across) and then build in twisting actions.

The final stage of rehabilitation is to use more intense racquet sport-based exercise. Begin with slow 'clockface' training:

- Stand with the foot of your uninjured leg on a line crossing of the court.
- Slowly step forwards (12 o'clock).
- Step sideways to the right (3 o'clock).
- Step backwards (6 o'clock).
- Step sideways to the left (9 o'clock).

Continue this action, speeding up gradually and widening your stride until you are eventually performing a 'jump lunge' action. Repeat the movement standing on your injured leg. Once you have mastered this action you can introduce an element of surprise by having someone call out the times of the clockface randomly. This will work on your muscle reaction speed, and train the hamstrings for that sudden lunging action needed to reach for an unpredictable ball.

 KEY POINT

The hamstrings perform fast whipping actions during a game. Begin with slow static stretching and build to dynamic stretching exercises and game drills.

Swollen knee

When the knee suffers a minor injury, it swells and limits the movement of the joint. As the swelling clots and the injury heals, movements will feel stiff and the knee may give way if it is unable to straighten completely. For this reason you need to work both the bending (flexion) and straightening (extension) movements of the knee. From these relatively simple movements you can finally progress to agility-based actions involving twisting, which also help to build confidence in the knee. This latter feature is often overlooked, but it is very important, especially if the knee has been giving way.

Of all sports, racquet sports place one of the greatest stresses on the knee, because they involve twisting on a fixed foot. The foot is firmly planted on the ground fixed by your body weight, while you move for a shot and turn your body. The meeting point of these two actions is the knee joint!

Begin your rehab programme using the rectus femoris stretch (I.2), but instead of pulling the thigh backwards level with the hip, allow the thigh to move forwards to take the stretch away from the muscles and re-direct it to the joint. To work on straightening, use exercise II.5, stretching the hamstrings with a towel. Again, re-focus the exercise by allowing the thigh to move downwards, so as to release the hamstring stretch and focus instead on locking the knee out fully. Once you are confident with these actions, move on.

 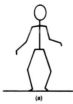 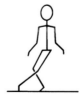 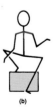

Developing agility in the knee: (a) grapevine movement to place sideways strain on the knee; (b) increasing range of movement

For the next movement, try the following:

- Stand with your feet shoulder width apart.
- Step forwards and across with the uninjured leg so that the stress is taken on the injured knee.
- Step backwards and across to place the opposite stress on the joint – see (a) in the diagram.

This action can be used as a side-step to perform a 'grapevine' action, stepping first in front and then behind the injured leg. Bending the knee further will increase the stress on the knee, and performing the action over a bench to bend the knee to near maximum will test the knee fully – see (b) in the diagram. Be cautious, however, because these actions stress the knee considerably, so they must be carefully controlled. You are now working for stretch, strength and balance of the knee all at the same time (agility). Using the clockface exercise described above (page 69) will also work the knee and prepare it for competition.

Groin strain

Groin strain is a common injury, often caused when you perform a wide lunging action during a game and stretch too far. There are two types of groin muscles, or adductors – the long adductors travel from the groin right down to the knee, and the short adductors go from the groin to the upper thigh only. Two exercises are useful for this area, one for the short adductor muscles and the other for the long.

Hip adductor stretches for groin strain

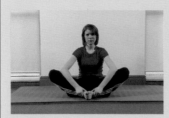

In the first exercise, begin by sitting on the floor with the soles of your feet together. Holding your feet with both hands, press down on your knees or thighs to push them apart.

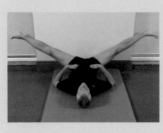

The second stretch (similar to exercise III.1) emphasises the long adductor:
• Lie on your back with your legs straight against a wall.
• Part your legs as far as possible.
• Allow your legs to lower slowly and hold this position.

In both exercises, contract–relax (CR) stretching may be used (see page 20). For this, apply resistance while lifting your legs (press down on your knees in the first stretch, and lift against gravity in the second). Hold the tensed position for 5–10 seconds and then lower your legs again to increase the stretch still further.

It is important when you are rehabilitating after groin strain that strength training and stretching go hand in hand. As the stretching feels easier, use dynamic movements. This can be done in a swimming pool with breaststroke-type actions, or in the gym using elastic tubing. When you get back on court, spend a few sessions practising rehab before you play. Use repeated side-step drills, zigzag running up and down court, backward running and diagonal runs across court. Vary the speed, step width and intensity, making sure you are pain free and confident before you play.

The calf and Achilles

When the Achilles tendon is injured, you should perform calf
stretches with your knee flexed (see exercise 1.3). When the calf is
injured, however, it is usually the long calf muscle (gastrocnemius)
that is affected, and you should stretch with the knee straight.

When you can perform this statically without pain, use the
exercise shown below.

As you return to racquet sports, use gentle jogging actions to
begin with and build up to side-stepping and zigzag runs across
court. Finally, practise lunges, pushing off from the injured foot.
Begin slowly and build up speed until you are confidently using
explosive lunges in multiple directions.

Calf and Achilles stretch

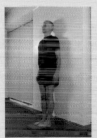

- Stand on a 5 cm block (a thick book or
  yoga block) and place the ball of your
  foot on the back edge.
- Allow the heel to lower, keeping the
  knee locked – this will stretch the long
  calf muscle.
- Starting from standing again, raise up
  on to your toes against your body weight.

Initially, you should hold onto something
to take some of your body weight off the calf. Eventually, you
can use your full body weight and speed up the exercise
until you are using faster, more explosive actions to work the
muscle intensely.

Catching shoulder

Catching shoulder (shoulder impingement) is a common injury in racquet sports. It occurs when a structure (usually one of the deep 'cuff' muscles of the shoulder) becomes trapped between the moving ball and socket of the shoulder joint. Normally there is a good clearance between the ball and socket, but this can be lessened through postural changes around the shoulder. Typically, a round-shouldered position, combined with tightness in the muscles that twist the arm inwards (shoulder medial rotators), pulls the ball of the shoulder forwards relative to the socket, so increasing the likelihood of catching.

There are two exercises you can use to address this postural tightness, one to stretch the tight chest (pectoral muscles) and one to twist the shoulder.

If one or both shoulders have been catching for some time you may have developed a 'limp' in your shoulder with the shoulder blade 'hitching' as you move your arm sideways. Look at yourself in a mirror as you lift your arm out sideways. Try to keep your shoulder level as your arm is lifted, avoiding any shrugging action. Repeat this action while holding your racquet, focusing on correct shoulder alignment as you do so.

If you find it difficult to spot any alignment change, go to a Pilates class for a couple of sessions and ask the instructor to watch you as you move your shoulder.

Tennis elbow

Tennis elbow is one of the best-known racquet sports injuries, although it is also very commonly caused by other repetitive activities such as hammering and using spanners. The problem occurs because the muscles on the back of the forearm (extensors)

Anterior chest and shoulders

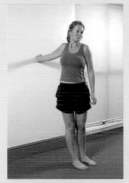

This exercise will stretch both the chest muscles and the front of the shoulder. Standing side on to a wall, place the hand of your affected arm on the wall at shoulder height. Keeping your arm straight, turn your feet in the opposite direction and rotate your body this way as well – so if your right arm is affected, turn your feet and body to the left. You will feel the stretch across the front of your affected shoulder. Keep the trunk twist slow and controlled.

Perform this as a static stretch, gradually building up the holding time from three–five seconds to 20–30 seconds. Aim to perform three reps, holding for 20–30 seconds every other day.

External shoulder rotation

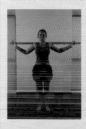 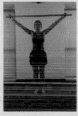

This exercise stretches the twisting muscles of your shoulder (rotator cuff). Grip a bar above your head, lower your arms so that the bar passes behind your neck, hold the position and then release. (You can use a towel instead of the bar, but make sure you keep it taut.) Build up the holding time as for the exercise above.

become tight, causing inflammation where they attach to a point of bone on the outside of the forearm. The result is aching over the outside of the forearm, with severe pain just on the point. This hurts when you grip a racquet, but also with seemingly innocuous day-to-day activities like picking up a mug of tea.

The muscles must be stretched by bending (flexing) the wrist while keeping the elbow complexly locked out. If you allow your elbow to bend even slightly, the stretch will be taken off, and the effect lost. The simple wrist extensor exercise (II.8) can help – performed correctly, this stretch can be felt as a gnawing sensation up the whole arm and into the elbow.

One of the muscles involved also pulls the wrist joint outwards (abduction), so a further stretch can be placed on this muscle by pulling your wrist inwards (adduction) at the same time as bending it. You can achieve this with the exercise, shown below.

Tennis elbow often involves the nerves travelling through the elbow as well. If this is the case you may feel pins and needles shooting into your fingers. See a physiotherapist to have the trapped nerve released.

Stretching the wrist muscles for tennis elbow

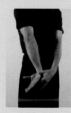

- Stand with your arm by your side.
- Twist the forearm downwards.
- Bend your wrist.
- Take hold of your hand and bend the wrist further, pulling it towards the little finger side.

Getting the balance right

Remember that the use of stretching for sports injuries should be *progressive*. This means that as you heal, you can stretch that little bit further or move a little faster. However, always bear in mind that this is a balance. You must do enough to help your body heal correctly, but not too much, in case you tear the healing tissues. Let pain be your guide here. If a stretch causes slight aching, that is fine, but if you feel pain, stop, rest and re-start the next day.

Remember also that racquet sports are highly skilled, so you must redevelop some of your former skill base following injury. For example, after a knee injury the exercise progression used should involve strength, stretching and speed. This will give you back your former fitness. The icing on the cake, however, is skill. Once you have your fitness back, ease yourself back into the game slowly. Begin by going on court by yourself and simply performing slow and then faster pace single shots, building to multiple sequences in varying directions

5

Training Log

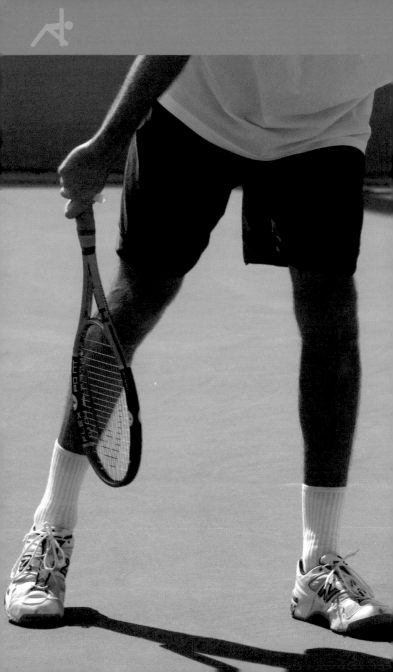

5. Training log

Phase I – Beginner   Use these tables to chart your progress. Refer to page 4 for guidance.

	Exercise	Average	Initial flexibility Less/average/more	Week 1 No of reps/sets performed	Week 1 Less/average/more	Week 2 No of reps/sets performed	Week 2 Less/average/more	Week 3 No of reps/sets performed	Week 3 Less/average/more
1	Hamstrings – active knee extension	Knee 23° short of fully locked							
2	Rectus femoris stretch – standing	Heel 10 cm from buttock							
3	Calf Lunge	Knee mid foot							

	Exercise	Average	Initial flexibility	Week 1		Week 2		Week 3	
			Less/ average/ more	No of reps /sets performed	Less/ average/ more	No of reps /sets performed	Less/ average/ more	No of reps /sets performed	Less/ average/ more
4	Thoracic spine – kneeling	Arms nearly in straight line with spine							
5	Spinal rotation – lying	Knee 10 cm from floor							
6	Hip flexors and extensors – modified lunge	Groin just above level of front knee							

Phase II – Intermediate

	Exercise		Average	Initial flexibility	Week 1		Week 2		Week 3	
				Less/ average/ more	No of reps /sets performed	Less/ average/ more	No of reps /sets performed	Less/ average/ more	No of reps /sets performed	Less/ average/ more
1	Anterior chest and shoulders		Upper arms 20° to body surface							
2	Lateral flexion – standing		Upper shoulder above groin							
3	Anterior tibials		Ankle 2.5 cm from ground							

	Exercise	Average	Initial flexibility	Week 1		Week 2		Week 3	
			Less/ average/ more	No of reps /sets performed	Less/ average/ more	No of reps /sets performed	Less/ average/ more	No of reps /sets performed	Less/ average/ more
4	Hip adductors – long sitting	Knee 15 cm from ground							
5	Knee extension – with towel	Knee nearly locked							
6	Hip flexors – Thomas test	Lower leg 10° above horizontal							

Exercise		Average	Initial flexibility	Week 1		Week 2		Week 3	
			Less/average/more	No of reps/sets performed	Less/average/more	No of reps/sets performed	Less/average/more	No of reps/sets performed	Less/average/more
7	Deep calf and Achilles	Knee over mid-foot							
8	Wrist extensors – against a wall	Back of wrist 2 cm from wall							

Phase III – Advanced

	Exercise	Average	Initial flexibility	Weeks 1/2		Weeks 2/3		Weeks 3/4	
			Less/ average/ more	No of reps /sets performed	Less/ average/ more	No of reps /sets performed	Less/ average/ more	No of reps /sets performed	Less/ average/ more
1	Hip adductors – wall support	90° angle between legs							
2	Gluteals	Hip held at 80° bend							
3	Hip flexors –supine lying	Upper leg 10 cm from chest							

Exercise		Average	Initial flexibility	Weeks 1/2		Weeks 2/3		Weeks 3/4	
			Less/ average/ more	No of reps /sets performed	Less/ average/ more	No of reps /sets performed	Less/ average/ more	No of reps /sets performed	Less/ average/ more
4	Hamstrings – swing on back	Straight leg 70° to vertical							
5	Leg swing – forwards and backwards	Leg 45° to horizontal							
6	Leg swing – sideways	Leg 30° to horizontal							

	Exercise	Average	Initial flexibility	Weeks 1/2		Weeks 2/3		Weeks 3/4	
			Less/ average/ more	No of reps /sets performed	Less/ average/ more	No of reps /sets performed	Less/ average/ more	No of reps /sets performed	Less/ average/ more
7	Calf stretch – sprint start	Back heel 5 cm from ground							
8	Shoulder rotation with towel	Fingers 10 cm apart							
9	Lying backwards trunk twist	Bent leg lowered to 15 cm above floor							

6

Terms you should know

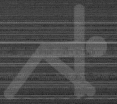

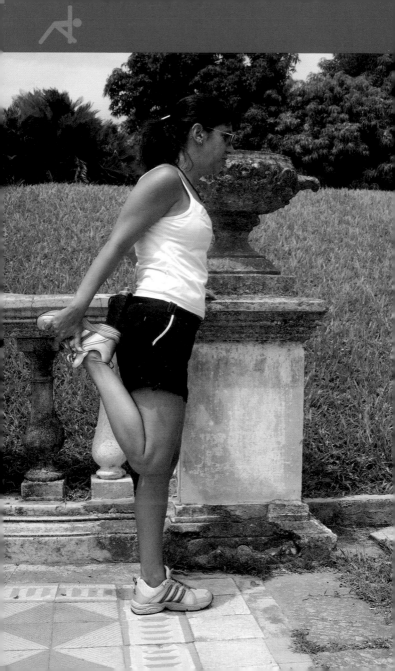

6. Terms you should know

Abduction – moving a limb away from you
Adduction – moving a limb in towards you
Agility – training which combines stretch, balance and strength
Arousal level – how 'psyched up' you are for exercise
Cardiovascular (CV) training – working your heart/lungs/circulation using exercise that makes you out of breath
Delayed onset muscle soreness (DOMS) – stiffness and soreness in muscles which occur one or two days after training
Dynamic stretch – stretching while moving
Extension – straightening a joint
Flexion – bending a joint
General exercise – exercise which works several body parts at once
Ischaemic muscle pain – 'the burn' felt during exercise, due to the build-up of muscle acids
Isolation exercise – exercise that focuses on a single body part
Isometric – a muscle contraction where you tense and hold
Lumbar spine – your lower back
Motivation – how keen you are to exercise
Movement range (or **range of motion**) – the amount of movement at a joint
Muscle fibre – each muscle is made up of thousands of microscopic fibres, arranged a little like the bristles on a shaving brush
Muscle imbalance – when one group of muscles is unnaturally stronger or more flexible than another
Overuse injury – one that comes on over time
Periodisation – a method of splitting your training programme up into sections so you do not practise all exercises in each workout
Pronation – turning the hand or foot downwards (palm to the floor or sole of the foot to the floor)
Repetition or rep – a single movement or exercise
Set – a group of repetitions, for example one set of five reps
Shin splint – pain in the muscles along the shin bones
Static stretch – stretch and hold
Training intensity – how hard you exercise

Training volume – how much exercise (numbers of sets and reps) you do
Traumatic injury – one that occurs suddenly
Treadmill – running road machine seen in gyms
Workout – the time you spend exercising